The Complete Keto Diet Lunch Cookbook

50 Inspired Recipes to Lose Weight and Stay Fit for Women Over 50

Katie Attanasio

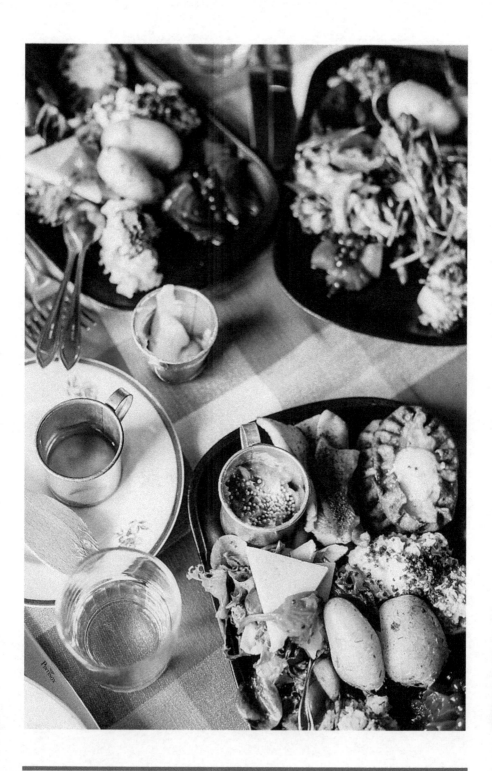

© Copyright 2021 - All rights reserved.

a result of the use of information contained within this document, including, but not limited to, — errors, omissions, or inaccuracies.

Table of Contents

50 Essential Lunch Recipes 8

1   Mediterranean Tuna Salad with Olives 8

2   Keto Green Bean Casserole 11

3   Keto Chicken Taco Soup 13

4   Crunchy Asian Cabbage Salad 15

5   Keto Dutch Baby with Chocolate and Macadamia 19

6   Parmesan Roasted Ranch Cauliflower with Avocado 21

7   Spinach Salad with Warm Bacon Dressing 23

8   Chicken Cobb Salad with Cobb Salad Dressing 25

9   Broccoli Cheddar Quiche with Bacon 26

10   Avocado Chicken Salad 28

11   Low Carb Chicken Soup 30

12   Sweet and Sour German Green Beans with Bacon and Onions 32

13   Thai Chicken Satay with Peanut Sauce 34

14   Fajita Hasselback Chicken 37

15   Chicken Spinach Blueberry Salad with Parmesan Cheese 39

16   Keto Tuna Melt 41

17   Cheesy Baked Zucchini Casserole 43

18   Mexican Keto Meatballs 45

19   Meat Lovers' Keto Stuffed Peppers 46

20   Instant Pot Short Ribs 48

21   Cheesy Artichoke Chicken Bake 50

22   Keto Club Sandwich 52

23   Keto Antipasto Salad 54

24   Zucchini Soup 56

25   Grilled Shrimp Citrus Marinated.. 58

26   Taco Zucchini Boats 60

27   Keto Buffalo Chicken Cauliflower Casserole................................. 62

28   Creamy Asparagus Soup 64

29   Low Carb Sausage And Kale Soup 66

30   One Pot Low Carb Sausage And Riced Veggies 68

31   Sriracha Grilled Leg Of Lamb 70

32   Tandoori Grilled Lamb Chops 72

33   Low Carb Meatball And Vegetable Casserole 74

34   Jalapeno Chicken And Broccoli Casserole 76

35   Bacon Cheddar Egg Salad 78

36   Sheet Pan Lemon Chicken And Asparagus 80

37   Curried Chicken Salad.. 82

38   Memphis BBQ Sausage And Cheese Platter.................................... 84

39   Keto Fideo 86

40   Loaded Baked "Potato" Soup 88

41   Texas Style Keto Venison Chili..91

42   Keto Mexican Street Cauliflower Salad 93

43   Keto Mexican Spaghetti Casserole... 95

44   Keto Zucchini Gratin with Poblanos...97

45   Keto Shrimp Etouffee with Crawfish 99

46   Keto Lemon & Garlic Grilled Chicken Quarters 101

47   Grilled Salmon with Cilantro Lime Crema 103

48   Mexican Shredded Beef 105

49   Chipotle Lime Grilled Pork Chops 107

50   Asian Inspired Ground Venison Lettuce Wraps 109

50 Essential Lunch Recipes

1   Mediterranean   Tuna   Salad   with Olives

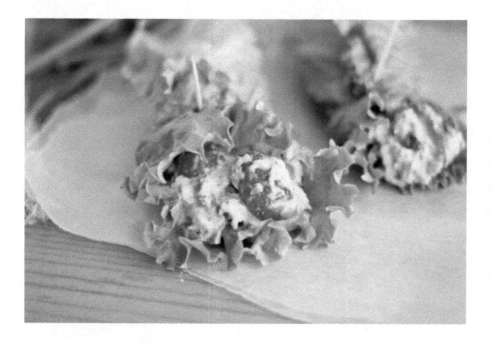

Servings: 1 | **Time:** 10 mins | **Difficulty**: Easy

Nutrients per serving: Calories: 351 kcal | Fat: 20g | Carbohydrates: 13.2g | Protein: 35.2g | Fiber: 2.9g

---

Ingredients

1 & 1/2 tsp Lemon juice, or to taste

1 Can Tuna, packed in water (5 oz. Drained)

1 Tbsp Paleo Mayo

1 Tbsp Sun-Dried Tomatoes Packed in Olive Oil, drained and diced

1 tsp Lemon zest

1 tsp Pine nuts

1/2 tsp Dried parsley

1/4 tsp Dried Basil

1/4 tsp dried oregano

2 Tbsp Roasted red peppers, sliced

4 Cherry Tomatoes, diced

4 Kalamata olives, sliced

Salt, to taste

Method

1.   Take oven to 350 °F.

2.   On a small baking sheet, cook around 5-7 minutes until the pine nuts turn to a light brown color. Don't burn them.

3.   Put all ingredients in the mug and stir. Use salt as seasoning and taste with lemon juice.

4. Chop and mix the pine nuts into the tuna.

5. Serve in wraps of lettuce or on toast.

2   Keto Green Bean Casserole

Servings: 6 | **Time:** 50 mins | **Difficulty**: Easy

Nutrients per serving: Calories: 159 kcal | Fat: 11g | Carbohydrates: 10.3g | Protein: 6.2g | Fiber: 3.3g

Ingredients

1 1/4 tsp. Sea salt

1 cup Onion, diced

2 cups Green beans, trimmed

1/3 cup 2% milk (or 1/2 cup almond milk)

1/4 Cup Full fat cream cheese (dairy-free works too)

1/4 tsp. Pepper

2 Cups Mushrooms, sliced

2/3 cup Half and half cream (or 1/2 cup full-fat coconut milk)

6 Slices Bacon

Method

1.   Heat the oven to 350 °F .

2.   Take a frying pan over medium heat.

3.   Cook until the bacon turns to golden brown color and crispy on sides.

4.   Then remove excess fat after transferring it to a paper towel. Reserve only 1 Tbsp. of fat.

5.   Add onions & mushrooms in a medium to high heated pan.

6.   Cook until golden brown by stirring sporadically for about 3 minutes.

7.   Boil all ingredients except beans.

8.   Boil for 4 minutes until the mixture thickens by stirring continuously.

9.   Cook by stirring continuously on reduced heat, and cook until mixture is very thick, for 7-8 minutes.

10.   Boil salted water in a large pot. Cook green beans until they become fork tender. It should take 7-8 minutes. Dry them by draining excess water and patting them with a paper towel.

11.   Then, add cooked beans into the sauce and stir to coat beans with sauce.

12.   Put into a pan of size 8x8 inch and cook for 15-20 minutes.

13.   While you are cooking beans, make crumbs of bacon in a food processor. Use casserole to sprinkle and bake for 5 minutes.

3   Keto Chicken Taco Soup

Servings: 4 | **Time:** 25 mins | **Difficulty:** Easy

Nutrients per serving: Calories: 215 kcal | Fat: 10.62g | Carbohydrates: 10.75g | Protein: 16.2g | Fiber: 2.1g

Ingredients

shredded cheddar cheese optional fresh sliced

jalapeno optional

8 oz full-fat cream cheese room temperature

4 tbsp fresh chopped cilantro optional

3 tbsp Low Carb Taco Seasoning

3 cups chicken broth

1 lime, cut into wedges optional

2 cups chicken breast tenders

1 cup of salsa

Method

1.   Take an instant pot and put the chicken broth, taco seasoning, and chicken in it.

2.   Make sure that the release valve is sealed. Choose a cycle time of about 15 minutes in manual mode. The cycle will start automatically.

3.   Once the cycle is completed, let it for 10 minutes. Then release the valve.

4.   Take chicken out of the pot and use a fork to shred it.

5.   Choose sauté setting on the instant pot.

6.   Whisk the cream with chicken broth mixture.

7.   Simmer the shredded chicken in the pot for about 3-4 minutes.

8.   If desired, top with cilantro, cheddar cheese shredded, lime wedge, and jalapeno.

4   Crunchy Asian Cabbage Salad

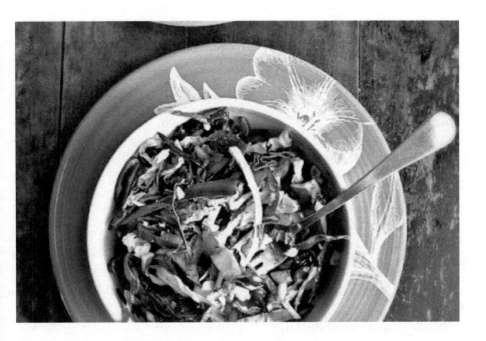

Servings: 4 | **Time:** 50 mins | **Difficulty:** Easy

Nutrients per serving: Calories: 519 kcal | Fat: 52g | Carbohydrates: 10g | Protein: 2.2g | Fiber: 2.9g

Ingredients

For Salad Dressing:

1 tsp Bragg's Amino Acids

1 tsp Dijon Mustard

2 tbsp Rice Wine Vinegar

1/4 cup Coconut Oil Liquid

Cabbage

Cucumbers

1/4 tsp Freshly Cracked Pepper

3 tbsp Rice Wine Vinegar

1/2 head Green Cabbage Cored and finely shredded

1/2 tsp Kosher Salt

1/2 cup Coconut Oil Liquid

1/4 cup Cilantro Chopped with no stems

1/2 Hothouse Cucumber Seeded

1 tbsp Sesame Seeds (Optional)

1/4 Fresh Red Chili Pepper (Optional) Sliced thin

1/4 tsp Kosher Salt

1 tbsp Olive Oil

Red peppers (Asian)

2 tsp Sesame Oil

1 Red Pepper cored, seeded, and sliced very thin

1/2 tsp Ginger Fresh, from a jar or 1/4 tsp dried ginger

1/4 cup Scallion Greens Sliced or 1/4 tsp Ground Cumin

2 tbsp finely diced shallots.

Remaining Ingredients:

1 Avocado Peeled, sliced and seeded

1 cup Snow Pea Pods

Optional Quick Pickled Onions

2 tbsp Red Wine Vinegar

1/4 cup Red Onion Finely diced

Asian cabbage

Method

1.   Take a large bowl and shred the cabbage in it. Mix well after adding the remaining ingredients.

2.   Don't let it sit at the bottom. Asian cucumbers

1.   Take a medium bowl and slice cucumbers in it.

2.   Put rest of the ingredients and rest it for 30 minutes. Asian red peppers

1.   Take a medium bowl and slice red peppers in it.

2.   Put rest of the ingredients and rest it for 30 minutes. Quick Pickled Onions

1.   Take a medium bowl and diced onions in it.

2.   Take red wine vinegar and cover the onions with it.

3.   Rest it for 20 minutes.

Salad Dressing:

1.   Take a bowl and add all the ingredients.

2.   Set it aside at room temperature after mixing. Cabbage Salad

1.   After marinating all the ingredients of the salad, put the cabbage in a bowl.

2.   Top it with equal portions of marinated red peppers, marinated cucumber, and sliced avocado. (In the case of snow peas, put peas into the salad.)

3.   Whereas, in the case of pickled onions, top them with a pinch of cilantro.

4.   And to garnish, use sesame seeds.

5 Keto Dutch Baby with Chocolate and Macadamia

Servings: 4 | **Time:** 20 mins | **Difficulty**: Easy

Nutrients per serving: Calories: 272 kcal | Fat: 23.62g | Carbohydrates: 8.74g | Protein: 8.52g | Fiber: 5.7g

Ingredients

4 large eggs

2 tbsp coconut flour

2 tbsp butter

1/8 tsp salt

1/4 cup monk fruit sweetener

1/4 cup heavy whipping cream

1/4 cup almond flour

1/2 cup sugar-free whipped cream optional

1/2 cup strawberries optional

1 tsp vanilla extract

1 tbsp sugar-free chocolate syrup

Method

1. Preheat the oven to 400 °F .

2. Put butter (2 tbsps.) in a preheated oven.

3. In a large bowl, whisk together 1/4 cup Sweetener (Monk fruit), 2 tbsp coconut flour, 1/8 tsp salt, and 1/4 cup almond flour.

4. In a second bowl, add 1 tsp vanilla extract, 4 large eggs, and 1/4 cup heavy whipped cream.

5. Stir until well combined.

6. Combine mixtures of egg and almond flour.

7. Remove skillet from the oven and pour batter (Dutch Baby) in skillet.

8. Bake skillet in the oven for 15 minutes to brown the Dutch Baby top.

9. Take 1 tbsp. ChocZero syrup and drizzle the pancake.

10. Take 1 tbsp. nuts (macadamia) and sprinkle the pancake.

11. Serve with fresh strawberries and sugar-free whipped cream.

6   Parmesan   Roasted   Ranch Cauliflower with Avocado

Servings: 4 | **Time:** 35 mins | **Difficulty**: Easy

Nutrients per serving: Calories: 179 kcal | Fat: 14.5g | Carbohydrates: 11g | Protein: 5g | Fiber: 6.5g

Ingredients

2 Tbsp. Olive oil

2 cups Cauliflower, cut into large florets

1 large avocado, cubed

2 Tbsp. Finely grated Parmesan cheese

2 Tbsp. Ranch mix (recipe below) Pinch of sea salt

Ranch Seasoning:

3/4 tsp Salt

1 Tbsp Dried Parsley

1 tsp Garlic powder

1/3 tsp Pepper

1 tsp Onion powder

1 tsp Dried Dill

Method

1.   Preheat the oven to 400 °F .

2.   Take a bowl, mix the oil and cauliflower in it.

3.   Add 2 Tbsp. of mixed ranch mix to cauliflower. Coat by tossing.

4.   Spread a single layer of cauliflower on a baking sheet. Leave space between the flowers.

5.   First, cook for 15 minutes and then cook again for 12 minutes after stirring until the color changes to Golden Brown.

6.   Toss with avocado, cheese, and some salt in a bowl.

7 Spinach Salad with Warm Bacon Dressing

Servings: 4 | **Time:** 30 mins | **Difficulty**: Easy

Nutrients per serving: Calories: 445 kcal | Fat: 32g | Carbohydrates: 5.14g | Protein: 28g | Fiber: 1.8g

Ingredients

2 oz Mushrooms, sliced very thinly (about 4 large)

10.5 oz Baby Spinach

4 large boiled eggs, chopped

8 oz Bacon, diced

Warm Bacon Dressing:

1/4 cup bacon grease

2 tbsp Red wine vinegar

1 tbsp Low carb brown sugar

2 tbsp Shallot, finely chopped

Salt and pepper to taste

1/2 tsp Dried tarragon

1 tbsp Whole Grain Mustard

Customize:

Mandarin oranges, apple, walnuts, strawberries, shrimp, blue cheese

Method

1.   Put diced bacon in a pan on medium heat.

2.   Cook for 5-6 minutes by stirring sporadically.

3.   Pour bacon oil into a small bowl after removing it from the pan.

4.   Chop or slice the eggs, mushrooms, and shallot.

5.   Heat mushrooms in a pan over medium heat to lightly cook them.

6.   Take shallots and sauté them.

7.   Turn the heat to medium-low and add the Sukrin Gold, bacon oil, tarragon, vinegar, and whole grain mustard. Combine all of these by stirring continuously.

8.   Add pepper and salt to taste.

9.   Toss the hot dressing with the spinach and divide between 4 serving bowls. Taste to adjust seasoning. Top with bacon, eggs, and mushrooms.

8   Chicken Cobb Salad with Cobb Salad Dressing

Servings: 2 | **Time:** 20 mins | **Difficulty**: Easy

Nutrients per serving: Calories: 632 kcal | Fat: 54g | Carbohydrates: 9.5g | Protein: 29g | Fiber: 5g

Ingredients

4 oz cooked chicken breast, diced (about 1 medium breast)

180 grams romaine lettuce, chopped (2 hearts of romaine)

2 large boiled eggs, quartered, sliced, or chopped

6 tbsp Cobb Salad Dressing (or blue cheese dressing)

2 oz cheddar cheese, cubed

4 slices cooked bacon, crumbled

2-3 green onions, sliced

1/2 Hass avocado, cubed or sliced

Method

1.   Take lettuce and toss it with cobb salad dressing.

2.   Divide it into 2 bowls.

3.   Serve

9   Broccoli Cheddar Quiche with Bacon

Servings: 6 | **Time**: 50 mins | **Difficulty:** Easy

Nutrients per serving: Calories: 457 kcal | Fat: 40g | Carbohydrates: 3.8g | Protein: 20g | Fiber: 0.5g

Ingredients

1/4 cup almond milk (or water)

6 large eggs

1/4 cup raw onions, finely chopped (1 ounce)

1 1/4 cup heavy cream

2 cups shredded cheddar cheese (8 ounces)

1/4 tsp salt

6 oz bite-sized broccoli florets (steamed until crisp-tender)

1/4 tsp white pepper

4 slices cooked bacon, crumbled

Method

1.   Preheat oven to 350 °F .

2.   Spray a baking spry on a 10″ plate.

3.   Cook the bacon and crumble it.

4.   Now, steam broccoli. And dice onions.

5.   Layer the ingredients on a quiche plate: 1/3 each of the broccoli, onion, 1/4 of the cheese, and bacon.

6.   Add the almond milk, heavy cream, salt, eggs, and pepper to a medium bowl and use a hand mixer to beat it.

7.   Then, take custard and pour over the quiche ingredients.

8.   Bake it for 40 minutes to brown the top.

9.   Serve.

10   Avocado Chicken Salad

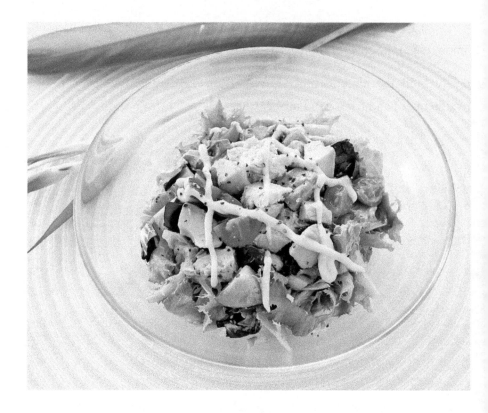

Servings: 3 | **Time:** 15 mins | **Difficulty**: Easy

Nutrients per serving: Calories: 267 kcal | Fat: 20g | Carbohydrates: 4g | Protein: 19g | Fiber: 1g

Ingredients

1 medium Hass Avocado, mashed

2 cups poached chicken diced (10 oz)

1/3 cup celery, finely diced (1 large rib)

2 tbsp cilantro, finely chopped

salt and pepper to taste

2 tbsp red onion or scallion, minced

1 tbsp fresh lemon juice (or lime juice)

2 tbsp avocado oil (or your favorite)

Method

1.   Prepare the onion, celery, and cilantro in a bowl.

2.   Take diced chicken and vegetables in the bowl.

3.   Cut avocado in half.

4.   Then scoop the flesh from the avocado.

5.   Use a fork to mash it and turn it to smoot and creamy texture.

6.   Take oil and lemon juice and stir the ingredients.

7.   Add all ingredients together in a bowl and mix by stirring.

8.   Serve with lettuce.

11 Low Carb Chicken Soup

Servings: 6 | **Time:** 30 mins | **Difficulty:** Easy

Nutrients per serving: Calories: 274 kcal | Fat: 15g | Carbohydrates: 8g | Protein: 26g | Fiber: 2g

Ingredients

6 cups bone broth

2 cups cooked chicken, diced Vegetable Base

1 cup celery, sliced

4 tbsp butter, avocado oil, or olive oil

1/2 cup onion, diced

1 large garlic clove, sliced 8 ounces celery root, cubed

1 whole bay leaf

1/3 cup carrot

2 tsp chicken base

1 tsp lemon zest

2 tsp lemon juice mixed with water

salt and pepper to taste

1 tbsp garlic herb seasoning blend

1/4 cup dry white wine

Method

1.   Take diced chicken.

2.   Take vegetables. Peel and cut them.

3.   Add butter, lemon zest, bay leaf, and vegetables in a quart pot on medium heat.

4.   Stir continuously to coat everything.

5.   Add chicken base, wine, and garlic herb blend after reducing the heat to medium.

6.   Cook vegetables for about 3-4 minutes until they turn brown.

7.   Boil the chicken broth, then simmer the vegetables over reduced heat until they become tender. Add the chicken broth and bring it to just under a boil.

8.   Add pepper and salt to taste.

12 Sweet and Sour German Green Beans with Bacon and Onions

Servings: 4 | **Time:** 18 mins | **Difficulty**: Easy

Nutrients per serving: Calories: 166 kcal | Fat: 11g | Carbohydrates: 8g | Protein: 9g | Fiber: 4g

Ingredients

4 slices bacon, diced

2 cups green beans

2 tbsp apple cider vinegar

1/4 cup onion, finely chopped

1 tbsp Low carb brown sugar

2 tbsp water

1 tsp wholegrain mustard

1/4 tsp salt

Method

1.   Take trimmed beans, chopped onions, and diced bacon.

2.   Turn beans tender by cooking.

3.   Cook bacon in a pan over medium heat for 4 minutes.

4.   Sauté the onions.

5.   Add the Sukrin Gold, water, onions, and cider vinegar to the bacon.

6.   Take a pan and put grain mustard in it.

7.   At last, take green beans and coat by stirring at heat thoroughly.

8.   Use pepper and salt to taste.

13 Thai Chicken Satay with Peanut Sauce

Servings: 4 | **Time**: 35 mins | **Difficulty:** Easy

Nutrients per serving: Calories: 279 kcal | Fat: 15g | Carbohydrates: 4g | Protein: 30g | Fiber: 1g

Ingredients

2 cups chicken tenders Chicken Satay Marinade

1 tbsp Hot Madras Curry Powder

1/3 cup full fat coconut milk from a can

1/4 cup chopped fresh cilantro (optional)

1/2 tsp ground coriander

2 tbsp Red Boat Fish Sauce (optional)

2 tbsp Low carb brown sugar

Peanut Sauce:

1/3 cup full fat coconut milk from a can

1 tsp soy sauce

1/4 cup smooth peanut/almond butter

1-2 tsp chile-garlic sauce

1 tbsp Low carb brown sugar

1/2 tsp Thai Red Curry Paste

Extras:

soaked bamboo skewers lime wedges

chopped fresh cilantro

Method

1.   take warm water and soak the skewers in it.

2.   Cut the chicken in half and place it in zip-lock bags.

3.   Take the satay marinade in a bowl and put a chicken in it to coat all sides of the chicken.

4.   Marinate overnight or for 30 minutes.

5.   Warm peanut butter in a small bowl.

6.   Whisk in the chile-garlic sauce, Sukrin Gold, Thai curry paste, and soy sauce.

7.   Then, add coconut milk slowly.

8.   Season it to taste.

9.   Refrigerate it.

10.   Thread the chicken tenders onto the bamboo skewers.

11. Cook the chicken on the grill, either indoor or outdoor.

12. Garnish it with fresh cilantro (chopped).

13. Serve with the peanut sauce and a lime wedge.

14   Fajita Hasselback Chicken

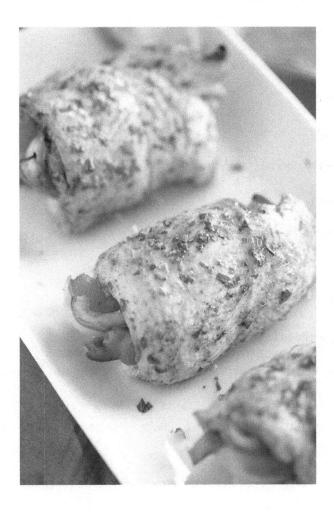

Servings: 4 | **Time:** 5 mins | **Difficulty:** Easy

Nutrients per serving: Calories: 368 kcal | Fat: 11g | Carbohydrates: 9g | Protein: 53g | Fiber: 1g

Ingredients

½ red bell pepper, diced

4 chicken breasts

½ yellow bell pepper, diced

½ onion, diced

2 Tbsps. fajita spice mix

½ cup cheddar cheese (50 g), grated

3 Tbsps. salsa

½ green pepper, diced

Method

1.   Take the oven to 350°F.

2.   Cut and slice the chicken but not deep enough to keep the bottom intact.

3.   Take fajita mix, and mix the cooked onions and pepper on medium heat.

4.   Take salsa and stir in the mixture. Use cheese to sprinkle over it.

5.   Melt the cheese and mix all ingredients.

6.   Fill chicken slices with 1 tbsp of mixture.

7.   Bake the chicken in the oven for 20 minutes, and juice run through it.

15 Chicken Spinach Blueberry Salad with Parmesan Cheese

Servings: 2 | **Time**: 20 mins | **Difficulty**: Easy

Nutrients per serving: Calories: 519 kcal | Fat: 38g | Carbohydrates: 10g | Protein: 35g | Fiber: 4g

Ingredients

Chicken Spinach Blueberry Salad:

6 cups baby spinach (170 g)

8 ounces chicken tenders or chicken breast

4 cups fresh blueberries

Two slices of red onion (paper-thin)

2 cups shaved Parmesan cheese

1 cup sliced almonds (toasted or raw)

Balsamic Dressing:

1 tbsp red wine vinegar

1/4 cup extra light olive oil

1 tbsp balsamic vinegar

r

2 tsp minced red onion

1/2 tsp dijon mustard

1 tbsp water

1 pinch each salt and pepper

1/8 tsp dried thyme

1/2 tsp low carb sugar

Method

1.   Grill the chicken thoroughly. And cut it into small pieces.

2.   Take almonds, and minced the onions, and make the dressing (balsamic).

3.   Brown the almonds slightly in a frying pan. Cool it after removing it from the pan.

4.   Add all ingredients of the dressing and blend them well with a stick blender.

5.   Take spinach and arrange it evenly on two plates.

16 Keto Tuna Melt

Servings: 4 | **Time**: 15 mins | **Difficulty**: Easy

Nutrients per serving: Calories: 227 kcal | Fat: 14g | Carbohydrates: 3g | Protein: 21g | Fiber: 1g

Ingredients

3 Tbsps. Mayonnaise

1.5 cups Canned Tuna

¼ cup Sliced celery

1 Tbsp. Finely diced red onion

4 slices Cheddar Cheese

2 Tbsps. Dill pickle relish

¼ Tsp. Salt

4 Tomato slices from a large tomato

Method

1.   Take a bowl. Add and stir mayonnaise, tuna, celery, red onion, and dill relish.

2.   Sprinkle some salt on the tomato slices placed on a baking sheet.

3. Then, on each slice, add 1/4 of the tuna mixture.

4. Take slices of cheese to top each tomato slice.

5. Cook until cheese melts. It should take about 3-5 minutes.

6. Serve

17 Cheesy Baked Zucchini Casserole

Servings: 6 | **Time:** 45 mins | **Difficulty:** Easy

Nutrients per serving: Calories: 275 kcal | Fat: 21g | Carbohydrates: 7g | Protein: 13g | Fiber: 1g

Ingredients

2 Tbsps. Butter

4.5 cups (approximately) zucchini, large, sliced

1/4 inch thick

1/2 cups Onion, diced

1 Tsp. Salt

1/2 cups Parmesan Cheese, grated and divided

½ cup Heavy Cream

2 cloves garlic, minced

1/2 cups Gruyere Cheese, grated and divided

Method

1.   Heat the oven to 450°F.

2.   Prepare and pace the salted zucchini slices on a paper towel.

3.   Let sit each side for 15 minutes each.

4.   Put zucchini slices on a dish.

5.   Take a skillet and heat the butter to melt it.

6.   Then add onion and garlic to cook them for 3 minutes and 2 minutes, respectively.

7.   Add the heavy cream while stirring in a pan.

8.   Add Gruyere cheese and Parmesan cheese and melt the cheese while stirring.

9.   Add the sauce (cheese) to the zucchini.

10.   Bake zucchini with parmesan and Gruyere for 5 minutes by covering the casserole dish with a foil. Remove it when tender.

11.   Serve.

18   Mexican Keto Meatballs

Servings: 15 meatballs| **Time**: 50 mins | **Difficulty:** Easy

Nutrients per serving (2 meatballs): Calories: 220 kcal | Fat: 18g | Carbohydrates: 2g | Protein: 14g | Fiber: 2g

Ingredients

2 Tbsps. Chili Powder

2 Tsps. Salt

2 Tbsps. Cumin

2 cups Ground Beef

1/4 cup Jalapenos, finely diced

1 Egg

85 g Cheddar Cheese, shredded

Method

1.   Take oven to 400°F.

2.   Take a large bowl and mix every ingredient in it.

3.   Bake balls of 2-inch size after rolling meat in balls like shape.

4.   For 25-30 minutes, bake them on a sheet (baking).

19   Meat Lovers' Keto Stuffed Peppers

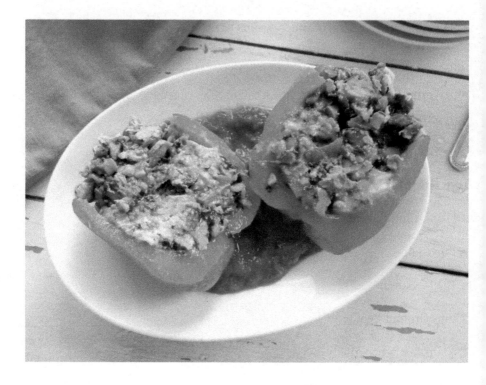

Servings: 6 | **Time**: 1 hr 10 mins | **Difficulty**: Easy

Nutrients per serving: Calories: 284 kcal | Fat: 22g | Carbohydrates: 6g | Protein: 16g | Fiber: 2g

Ingredients

225 g Mozzarella cheese

50 g Pepperoni small pieces

3 Bell peppers, any color

¾ cup Pasta sauce

Cooked 175 g Italian sausage

Method

1.   Heat oven to 400°F.

2.   Cut pepper and place them on the dish after removing seeds in them.

3.   On the bottom side of each pepper, put 1 tbsp. Sauce.

4.   Use pepperoni pieces and 30 g of Italian sausage as a topping.

5.   Put some mozzarella.

6.   Put sauce, pepperoni, and mozzarella again as the topping. Make sure to fill pepper with enough mozzarella.

7.   Bake peppers in the oven for 40 minutes until cheese is melted.

20   Instant Pot Short Ribs

Servings: 4 | **Time:** 2 hrs 30 mins | **Difficulty:** Easy

Nutrients per serving: Calories: 363 kcal | Fat: 21g | Carbohydrates: 4g | Protein: 33g | Fiber: 1g

Ingredients

Kosher salt

4 cups Short Ribs

1 Tbsp. Olive Oil Pepper

2 sprigs Rosemary

2 Bay Leaves

1 Onion, cut into quarters

4 sprigs thyme

3 large Carrots, cut into quarters

 2-4 cups Beef Broth

½ cup Red Wine

Method

1.   Put pepper and salt on all sides of the ribs.

2.   Add olive oil 1 tbsp. in the pot on sauté setting.

3.   Brown sides of ribs, it takes 2 minutes for each side.

4.   Set aside beef ribs.

5.   Cook onions and carrots in the pot for 5 minutes.

6.   Cook with red wine.

7.   Put herbs wrapped in cheesecloth with onions and carrots in a pressure cooker.

8.   Now, Put beef ribs in the pot.

9.   Take out the broth in another pot.

10.   For 1.5 hours, cook everything in a pressure cooker on high pressure.

11.   When done, release the pressure.

12.   Strain vegetables and beef in a bowl and put away herbs and vegetables.

13.   Serve.

21   Cheesy Artichoke Chicken Bake

Servings: 8 | **Time:** 1 hr. | **Difficulty**: Easy

Nutrients per serving: Calories: 399 kcal | Fat: 27g | Carbohydrates: 3g | Protein: 34g | Fiber: 1g

Ingredients

6 slices bacon, chopped and cooked

200 g Quartered artichoke hearts,

4 cups chicken breasts

1/4 c Mayonnaise

150 g Smoked Gouda

30 g Fresh baby spinach, chopped

1/2 Tsp. Onion powder

60 g Cream cheese, softened

85 g Havarti or Gruyere

1 Tsp. Garlic powder

Method

1.   Heat the oven to 400°F.

2.   Cut each chicken breast horizontally into two slices.

3.   Stir all ingredients together except chicken.

4.   Put the chicken in an oiled dish and use salt to sprinkle over it.

5.   Then, spread cheese on chicken.

6.   Put 4 breasts on cheese mixture.

7.   Bake in the oven for 30 minutes by covering with foil.

8.   Keep cooking until the chicken is cooked thoroughly.

22   Keto Club Sandwich

Servings: 2 | **Time:** 10 mins | **Difficulty**: Easy

Nutrients per serving: Calories: 413 kcal | Fat: 28g | Carbohydrates: 5g | Protein: 35g | Fiber: 1g

Ingredients

1 Tbsp. Mayonnaise

60 g Cheddar Cheese sliced

6 Iceberg lettuce leaves

180 g Deli Turkey sliced

2 slices Cooked Bacon

150 g Tomato slice

120 g Deli Ham sliced

Method

1.   Take out the core of iceberg lettuce.

2.   Peel off lettuce leaves.

3.   Spread mayonnaise on top of the two lettuce leaves.

4.   Put 30 g of cheese on the lettuce slice and use the deli ham slice as topping on leaves.

5.   Similarly, use two lettuce leaves to spread over the ham with mayonnaise. Top with sliced tomato, the cooked bacon, sliced deli turkey, and cheese.

6.   Again, use mayonnaise on turkey and put lettuce leaves on it.

7.   Cut in 4 pieces and put a toothpick in each piece.

23   Keto Antipasto Salad

Servings: 8 | **Time:** 1 day 25 mins | **Difficulty:** Easy

Nutrients per serving: Calories: 444 kcal | Fat: 36g | Carbohydrates: 10g | Protein: 19g | Fiber: 4g

Ingredients

250 g Prosciutto

1 head Cauliflower

250 g Genoa Salami

150 g Roasted red peppers

5-6 leaves Fresh Basil

90 g Pepperoncini

90 g Black olives

240 g Fresh mozzarella

410 g Artichoke Heart quatres, drained

Dressing:

2 Tsp. Garlic powder

1 cup Olive oil

2 Tsp. Dried oregano

1/2 cup Red wine vinegar

3/4 Tsp. Salt

1 Tsp. Onion powder

2 Tsp. Lemon juice

1/2 Tsp. Pepper

Method

1.   Whisk together all the dressing ingredients in a small cup.

2.   Cut cauliflower into bite-sized florets and position them with about 1 inch of water in a pot. Place the lid on the pot and bring the cauliflower to a boil for 3-5 minutes, steaming until slightly tender.

3.   Drain and pat the cauliflower and rinse. Place in a gallon-size resealable bag, and pour half of the dressing over it. Place it in the refrigerator for at least 1 hour or overnight to marinate.

4.   Toss all the ingredients together the next day and pour the rest of the dressing over the antipasto salad.

5.   Chill until it's ready for serving.

24 Zucchini Soup

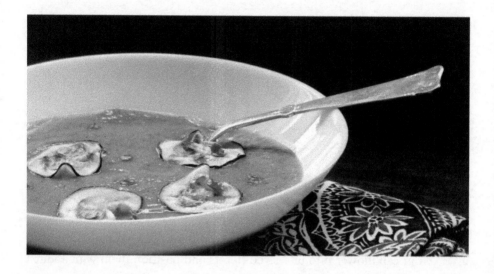

Servings: 8 | **Time:** 30 mins | **Difficulty:** Easy

Nutrients per serving: Calories: 64 kcal | Fat: 3g | Carbohydrates: 6g | Protein: 2g | Fiber: 1g

Ingredients

800 g Zucchini

¼ Tsp. Pepper

2 cloves Garlic

¼ cup Heavy cream

210 g sliced onion

½ Tsps. Kosher salt

400 g Chicken Broth

Method

1.   Place a lid on it and add the onion, garlic cloves, chicken broth, and zucchini to a large pot. Bring to a boil, then reduce heat to medium and let it simmer, occasionally stirring, for 20 minutes.

2.   Remove the pot from the heat until the zucchini is incredibly soft and use an immersion blender to combine it into a smooth puree.

3.   Using the puree to add salt and pepper and then mix in the heavy cream.

4.   Serving and loving!

25 Grilled Shrimp Citrus Marinated

Servings: 8 shrimp | **Time**: 30 mins | **Difficulty**: Easy

Nutrients per serving: Calories: 244 kcal | Fat: 3g | Carbohydrates: 4g | Protein: 46g

Ingredients

2 Tbsp. Orange zest

1 cup Olive oil

900 g Medium - Large shrimp

2 Tbsp. Lime zest

1/2 cup Orange Juice

2 Tbsp. Lemon zest

1/2 cup Lime juice

1/2 cup Lemon juice

1/2 Tsp. Ginger, grated

1/2 Tsp. Pepper

1/4 cup Cilantro

3 Tbsps. Garlic, minced

1/4 cup Parsley

1 Tsp. Salt

Method

1.   Combine the olive oil, zest, orange juice, lemon and lime juice, minced garlic, parsley, ginger, salt, cilantro, and pepper in a large cup. Together, whisk.

2.   Set to the side of 1/2 cup of the marinade.

3.   In a large freezer bag or airtight tub, put the shrimp and pour the leftover marinade on them. To coat, toss the shrimp and seal them in a jar or bag and put them in the refrigerator for 30 minutes - 1 hour to marinate.

4.   Take it out of the jar once the shrimp is marinated, avoiding any excess marinade when you put the shrimp on skewers. Dispose of the remaining marinade after skewering all the shrimp.

5.   Grill each side for 2-3 minutes or until the shrimp is pink and cooked.

6.   Until serving, drizzle the unused marinade over the cooked shrimp (no raw shrimp should have touched the marinade).

26   Taco Zucchini Boats

Servings: 8 | **Time:** 40 mins | **Difficulty:** Easy

Nutrients per serving: Calories: 242 kcal | Fat: 16g | Carbohydrates: 6g | Protein: 19g | Fiber: 1g

Ingredients

2 cups Ground beef

4 Zucchini

1 Tbsp. Chili Powder

¼ cup Water

½ cup Bell Peppers, mixed Red & Yellow

1/2 Tsp. Salt

2 Tsps. Cumin

1/2 cup Salsa

240 g Cheddar cheese, shredded

Method

1.   Preheat the oven to 400°F.

2.   Have your zucchini ready by cutting off the end of the stem.

3.   Place the zucchini boats and sprinkle a small amount of salt over them in a greased baking dish.

4.   Brown the ground beef in a skillet over medium heat.

5.   Connect the ground beef to the chili powder, bell peppers, salt, cumin, and 1/4 cup of water. Keep cooking until the vegetables are softened and water is absorbed.

6.   Fill each zucchini vessel with the beef and vegetable mixture until the beef mixture is ready.

7.   Top the vessels with zucchini and cheddar cheese.

8.   Bake for 20 minutes or until you have softened the zucchini and melted the cheese.

9.   Before serving, pour salsa over the boats.

27 Keto Buffalo Chicken Cauliflower Casserole

Servings: 8 | **Time:** 45 mins | **Difficulty**: Easy

Nutrients per serving: Calories: 372 kcal | Fat: 30g | Carbohydrates: 5g | Protein: 19g | Fiber: 1g

Ingredients

⅓ cup Frank's Red-Hot Sauce

520 g Cauliflower

¼ cup Ranch dressing

1 cup Celery, chopped

2 Eggs

250 g Cream Cheese, softened

240 g Cheddar cheese

350 g Chicken

Method

1.   Preheat the oven to 350°F.

2.   Remove the core from the head of your cauliflower and cut into bite-sized pieces.

3.   By sticking it in boiling water for 3 minutes or steaming in the microwave until it is fork-tender, blanch the cauliflower. Dry and set aside.

4.   Stir the hot sauce, ranch dressing, cream cheese, and eggs together in a big bowl.

5.   To the cream cheese mixture, add the cauliflower, 4 ounces of cheddar cheese, chicken, and celery and toss until well coated.

6.   Pour the remaining cheddar cheese into an 11x7 inch casserole dish and sprinkle with it.

7.   Bake for 30 minutes or until the cheese is melted and bubbly and the cauliflower is cooked.

28   Creamy Asparagus Soup

Servings: 8 | **Time:** 30 mins | **Difficulty**: Easy

Nutrients per serving: Calories: 110 kcal | Fat: 8g | Carbohydrates: 6g | Protein: 3g | Fiber: 2g

Ingredients

2 Tbsps. Butter

900 g Asparagus, trimmed

5 cups Chicken broth

1 Onion, thinly sliced

1-2 Tbsps. Lemon juice

Salt and pepper to taste

1/2 cup Heavy Cream

Method

1.   Break the asparagus and roughly chop the onion into 1-inch pieces.

2.   Heat a medium pot over medium-high heat with butter on the burner.

3.   Add the onion and asparagus and cook for 2 minutes.

4.   Add the broth and cover it with a lid, then boil.

5.   Reduce it to a simmer once it reaches a boil and cook for 20 minutes or until the vegetables are extremely tender.

6.   Remove the pot from the heat and puree the contents using a stick blender until it's smooth.

7.   Stir the cream in. Note: At this stage, you should add more broth until it has the perfect consistency, if the soup is thicker than you prefer.

8.   Connect the lemon juice and, to taste, salt and pepper.

29   Low Carb Sausage And Kale Soup

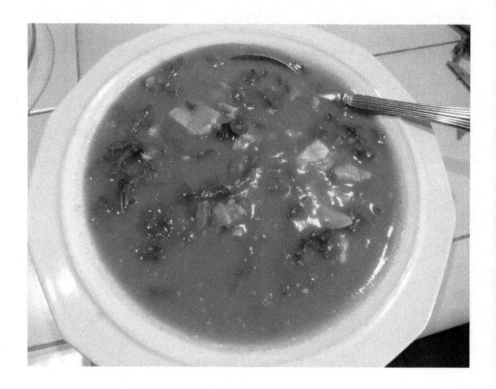

Servings: 6 | **Time**: 25 mins | **Difficulty:** Easy

Nutrients per serving: Calories: 164 kcal | Fat: 3g | Carbohydrates: 9g | Protein: 20g | Fiber: 3g

Ingredients

450 g Italian turkey sausage, sliced

960 g Chicken broth

1/2 cup Onion, diced

240 g Kale, stem removed

450 g Diced tomatoes

Method

1.   Set the Instant Pot to sauté the sausage.

2.   Turn off the Instant Pot and add to the pot the onions, diced tomatoes, and chicken broth.

3.   Fasten the cap and shut the steam valve on your Instant Pot or pressure cooker. Set to manual, high energy, 15 minutes.

4.   While the soup heats, put the chopped kale in a microwave dish with about 1/2 a cup of water.

5.   After the time is up, let the pressure cooker sit for about 10 minutes and then carefully open the valve to release the rest of the steam.

6.   Open the lid and add kale to your pressure cooker before serving.

30 One Pot Low Carb Sausage And Riced Veggies

Servings: 4 | **Time**: 20 mins | **Difficulty:** Easy

Nutrients per serving: Calories: 660 kcal | Fat: 60g | Carbohydrates: 7g | Protein: 13g | Fiber: 7g

Ingredients

120 g Onion

2 tbsp Olive oil

1.5 c Kale

Salt and pepper to taste

1 bag Green Giant Riced Cauliflower & Sweet Potato

1/4 c Goat cheese

4 cups Italian sausage

Method

1.   Apply the olive oil and the Italian sausage to a skillet over medium-high heat. For 5 minutes, cook.

2.   Add the diced onions to the pan and sauté them for another 5 minutes with the Italian sausage or until the sausage is cooked.

3.   Add the rice and vegetables and kale to cook for 5 minutes or until the kale and the riced veggies are tender and warmed up.

4.   To taste, apply salt and pepper.

5.   Serve and sprinkle with some goat's crumbled cheese.

31 Sriracha Grilled Leg Of Lamb

Servings: 10 | **Time:** 1 hr 10 mins | **Difficulty:** Easy

Nutrients per serving: Calories: 337 kcal | Fat: 23g | Carbohydrates: 2g | Protein: 32g

Ingredients

2 cloves Garlic

5 cups Leg of Lamb

1 tsp Paprika

2 Tbsp Sriracha

1/2 c Mayonnaise

1 tsp Salt

Method

1.   In a cup, combine salt, paprika, mayonnaise, garlic, and Sriracha, then dump into a freezer bag for a gallon.

2.   In the freezer bag, add a leg of lamb and rub it with the marinade. Seal the bag and put it in the refrigerator for at least 30 minutes, up to 4 hours, to marinate.

3.   Remove the lamb from the bag and put it on a grill that is 400 °F F. Sear for 5 minutes on either side.

4.   Close the grill lid and cook for 30-40 minutes or until the inside temperature of the lamb reaches 130°F F.

5.   Take it off the grill and let it rest for 10 minutes. Slice and serve.

32   Tandoori Grilled Lamb Chops

Servings: 2 | **Time:** 51 mins | **Difficulty:** Easy

Nutrients per serving: Calories: 475 kcal | Fat: 24g | Carbohydrates: 15g | Protein: 59g | Fiber: 2g

Ingredients

1 1/2 tbsp Garam masala

6 Lamb chops

3/4 c Greek yogurt

3 Garlic cloves, minced

2 tbsp Lemon juice

1 tbsp Turmeric

1 tsp Ginger, minced

1 tsp Salt

¼ tsp Cayenne Pepper

2 tsp Paprika

Method

1.   Combine the garlic, mayonnaise, paprika, salt, and Sriracha in a cup, then pour a gallon in a freezer bag.

2.   Rub a lamb leg with the marinade. Put it in the bag and refrigerate for 0.5-4 hours.

3.   Remove the lamb from the bag and place it on a 400°F grill.

4.   Sear on either side for 5 minutes.

5.   Close and cook the grill lid for 30-40 minutes or until the lamb's inside temperature reaches 130°F.

6.   Take it off the grill and leave for 10 minutes to rest. Slicing and serving.

33 Low Carb Meatball And Vegetable Casserole

Servings: 4 | **Time:** 30 mins | **Difficulty:** Easy

Nutrients per serving: Calories: 474 kcal | Fat: 39g | Carbohydrates: 10g | Protein: 25g | Fiber: 2g

Ingredients

1 c Eggplant

16 Cooked Perfect Fresh Meatballs

2 c Bell peppers

1 c Zucchini

1 c Squash

2 tbsp Olive oil

½ c Red onion, (diced)

240 g Fresh mozzarella

1 c Low carb pasta sauce

Salt and pepper to taste

Method

1.   In a wide bowl, put the diced vegetables and toss them in olive oil.

2.   To taste, apply salt and pepper.

3.   Spread low carb pasta sauce in a casserole dish and then add vegetables to spread them out evenly.

4.   Nestle meatballs with vegetables and top with fresh mozzarella bites.

5.   Cover the dish with foil and cook for 20 minutes in the oven at 350 ° F or until the vegetables are tender.

34 Jalapeno Chicken And Broccoli Casserole

Servings: 6 | **Time:** 45 mins | **Difficulty:** Easy

Nutrients per serving: Calories: 387 kcal | Fat: 27g | Carbohydrates: 7g | Protein: 31g | Fiber: 1g

Ingredients

240 g Cream cheese, softened

4-5 cups Chicken breast, cubed

½ c Heavy cream

½ c Parmesan, shredded

1 tsp Garlic powder

2 c fresh broccoli florets

1 tsp Onion powder

1 c Mozzarella, shredded

½ tsp Pepper

½ tsp Salt

1 Jalapeno, seeded & diced

Method

1.   In a big bowl, add the heavy cream, garlic powder, onion powder, cream cheese, salt and pepper.

2.   Add the jalapenos diced and stir until mixed.

3.   To the cheese mixture, add the cubed chicken and fold them together until the chicken is covered in the cheese.

4.   Spoon into a 13x9-inch baking dish that is greased.

5.   Florets of Nestle broccoli into the chicken.

6.   Mozzarella and Parmesan cheese topping.

7.   Cover and bake for 25 mins at 400°F. Uncover and bake for an extra 5 minutes.

35   Bacon Cheddar Egg Salad

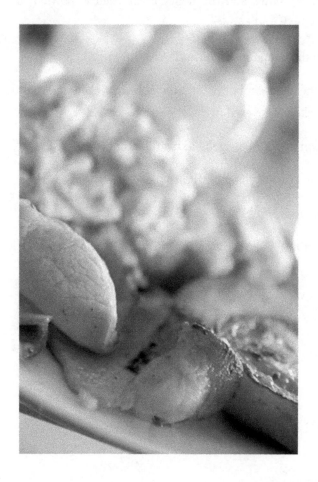

Servings: 6 | **Time:** 15 mins | **Difficulty**: Easy

Nutrients per serving: Calories: 458 kcal | Fat: 42g | Carbohydrates: 1g | Protein: 15g

Ingredients

Salt to taste

12 Hard-boiled eggs

1/2 cup Bacon, diced

1/2 cup Cheddar cheese, shredded and diced

1 Tbsp. Mustard

1 cup Mayonnaise

Method

1.   Take a large bowl and add chopped boiled eggs.

2.   Add mustard and mayonnaise, stir it.

3.   Add cheddar and bacon, fold mixture together.

4.   Salt to taste.

36 Sheet Pan Lemon Chicken And Asparagus

Servings: 4 | **Time:** 25 mins | **Difficulty:** Easy

Nutrients per serving: Calories: 272 kcal | Fat: 4g | Carbohydrates: 5g | Protein: 41g | Fiber: 2g

Ingredients

2 fresh lemons, sliced

5 ½ cups Chicken tenders

1 tsp Kosher salt

1 bunch Asparagus Olive oil

60 g Parmesan, shaved

2-3 Tbsp Lemon Pepper

Method

1.   Place the slices on a oiled baking sheet and slice the lemons into circles.

2.   Place the tender asparagus and chicken over the lemon slices.

3.   Drizzle it all with olive oil and sprinkle it with salt.

4.   Using lemon pepper to sprinkle the chicken tenders.

5.   Bake for 15-20 minutes at 425 °F or until the chicken is fully cooked.

6.   Shaved Parmesan garnish.

37   Curried Chicken Salad

Servings: 6 | **Time:** 20 mins | **Difficulty:** Easy

Nutrients per serving: Calories: 422 kcal | Fat: 33g | Carbohydrates: 6g | Protein: 29g | Fiber: 3g

Ingredients

1-2 tsp Curry Powder

5 ½ cups Chicken Breast

1/2 c Red Bell Pepper

Salt to taste

1 c Almonds

3/4 c Mayonnaise

CURRY POWDER:

2 Tbsp Ground Cumin

2 Tbsp Ground Cardamom

1/4 tsp Cayenne

1 Tbsp Ground Turmeric

1 Tbsp Dry Mustard

2 Tbsp Ground Coriander

Method

1.   Mix all the curry powder spices and store them in an airtight jar.

2.   Place in a wide bowl the sliced, cooked chicken breast and add the mayonnaise and the 1 Tsp. Curry powder, with a pinch of salt.

3.   Thoroughly mix and taste. Until you are pleased with the taste, continue adding curry powder and salt.

4.   Gently fold in and add the sliced almonds and diced red bell pepper.

5.   Store until ready to eat in the refrigerator.

38 Memphis BBQ Sausage And Cheese Platter

Servings: 8 | **Time:** 35 mins | **Difficulty**: Easy

Nutrients per serving: Calories: 660 kcal | Fat: 60g | Carbohydrates: 7g | Protein: 13g | Fiber: 7g

Ingredients

4 Tbsps. Stubb's Original BBQ Sauce

240 g Cheddar Cheese

10 Dill Pickles

1 Jar Pepperoncinis

2 cups Smoked Sausage

240 g Pepper Jack Cheese

Method

1.   Put the sausage on the heated grill and baste it with the Original BBQ Sauce.

2.   Put sausage on both sides and let it cook for about 10 minutes.

3.   Flip the sausage over when it is ready and proceed to cook.

4.   From the grill, detach the sausage and cut it into slices.

5.   Put the pepperoncini, pickles, cheese, and some more Stubb's sauce on a plate for dipping.

39   Keto Fideo

Servings: 4 | **Time:** 20 mins | **Difficulty**: Easy

Nutrients per serving: Calories: 409 kcal | Fat: 29g | Carbohydrates: 7g | Protein: 29g | Fiber: 4g

Ingredients

2 cups ground beef (or venison)

1/2 cup diced onion

1 tsp. salt

2 Tbsp. chili powder

3/4 cup chicken stock or bone broth

1 package of Palmini linguini, drained and rinsed

2 Tbsp. grated parmesan

1/3 cup grated mild cheddar

1 tsp. garlic powder

Method

1.   Start to brown the ground meat in a skillet over medium-high heat and use salt to season it.

2.   Cook until meat is browned and onions become translucent.

3.   First put palming drain and cook for 2 minutes then add chili and garlic and again cook for 1 minute.

4.   Cook for another 3 minutes and add cheese while stirring.

5.   Serve.

40 Loaded Baked "Potato" Soup

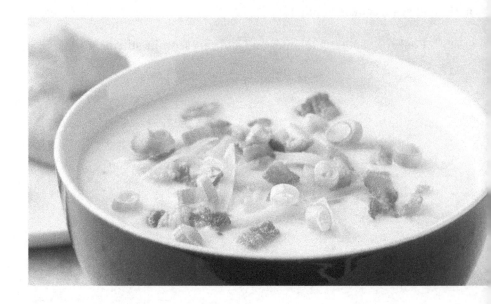

Servings: 5 | **Time:** 17 mins | **Difficulty:** Easy

Nutrients per serving: Calories: 204.97 kcal | Fat: 17.1g | Carbohydrates: 10.62g | Protein: 3.45g | Fiber: 3.26g

Ingredients

1/4 cup chopped onion

3 Tbsp. Butter

340 g bag frozen cauliflower

2 cups medium turnips

1 tsp. Salt

1 rib celery cut into 1" pieces

2 1/3 cups chicken broth

1/2 tsp. Garlic powder

Crispy bacon, crumbled

1/2 cup heavy cream

Sliced scallions or green onion

Cheddar cheese

2 Tbsp. Sour cream

Method

1.   Cook according to package instructions or steam the cauliflower until tender.

2.   In a medium saucepan over medium heat, melt the butter. Add the onions, diced celery and turnips. Season with garlic powder and salt and sauté until onions are translucent and turnips start to gather a little golden brown color and start to soften, around 7-10 minutes, over medium heat. Connect the cauliflower and continue cooking for 2-3 more minutes.

3.   Add the chicken stock to the vegetables and bring to a boil and reduce the heat for 5-7 minutes or until the turnips are fork-tender.

4.   Pour the vegetable and stock mixture into the mixer carefully. Apply the milk and sour cream and mix until creamy and smooth.

This is best achieved in a high-powered blender, but it can also work well in a conventional blender or immersion blender, although the texture might not be as smooth. When mixing hot liquids, use care and cover the top of the mixer with a towel. If you want a thinner soup, use some extra broth!

5.   If needed, taste and re-season with salt and pepper. Top and enjoy with bacon, cheese and green onion!

41   Texas Style Keto Venison Chili

Servings: 6 | **Time:** 1 hr | **Difficulty:** Easy

Nutrients per serving: Calories: 360 kcal | Fat: 19g | Carbohydrates: 10g | Protein: 36g | Fiber: 4g

Ingredients

3 1/3 cups ground venison or beef

3 Tbsps. Lard or bacon fat

1 bell pepper chopped

1/2 medium onion chopped

4 cloves garlic minced

3 Tsps. Garlic powder

1 poblano pepper seeded and chopped

1 Tbsp. Pepper

1 Tsp. paprika

2 Tbsps. Kosher salt

400 g cans diced tomato

2 Tbsps. chili powder

250 ml bottle low carb beer

Cups of water

3 Tbsps. tomato paste

1/2 Tbsp. cumin

Method

1. Combine the lard, fat, or oil with the ground meat in a big pot. 1 tsp kosher salt, 1/2 tsp pepper, and 2 tsp garlic powder season the beef. Cook ground meat until it is brown and caramelized over medium-high to high heat. Don't skip this move because it will give the chili an incredible depth of flavor.

2. Reduce the heat to medium-high and add the onion, peppers, and garlic, cooking for 5-7 minutes or until the vegetables soften. The vegetables will help deglaze the pan by picking up all of the browned meat pieces.

3. Combine the tomatoes, tomato paste, beer, water, and the remaining seasonings in a large mixing bowl.

4. Cover and cook for 30 minutes on medium, stirring occasionally. Remove the lid and continue to cook for another hour or so, until the meat is tender and the chili is the consistency you like. When the chili is simmering uncovered, it will reduce and thicken. Simply keep the cover on if you want a thinner chili. The longer you cook the chili, the more tender and decadent it becomes... I've had it on a low simmer on the stove all afternoon!

5. Serve with your favorite low-carb corn bread and a heaping helping of toppings!

42 Keto Mexican Street Cauliflower Salad

Servings: 12 | **Time**: 40 mins | **Difficulty:** Easy

Nutrients per serving: Calories: 152 kcal | Fat: 13g | Carbohydrates: 7g | Protein: 4g | Fiber: 2g

Ingredients

1 ½ tsp. salt

2 large heads fresh cauliflower cut into small florets

1/4 cup diced purple onion

1 tsp. garlic powder

4 Tbsp. avocado oil

2 Tbsp. chopped cilantro

1 cup cherry or grape tomatoes, halved

1 jalapeno

½ tsp. pepper

1/2 cup diced bell pepper

For the Dressing:

1/2 cup sour cream

1 Tbsp. fresh lime juice

¼ cup mayonnaise your favorite

1/4 tsp. paprika

1/3 cup + 2 Tbsp. crumbled Cotija cheese

1/2 tsp. cumin

¼ tsp. salt

2-3 cloves garlic finely minced

1/2 tsp. chili powder

Method

1.   Preheat to 425°F the oven. Using the salt, avocado oil, pepper and garlic powder to toss the florets and put the cauliflower florets on a lined sheet tray. For 20-25 minutes or until tender, roast at 425°F.

2.   Combine the cooled cauliflower, jalapeno, bell pepper, cabbage, tomatoes and coriander in a broad bowl and shake.

3.   Stir the mayo, sour cream, and the next 7 ingredients together. Combine the vegetables with the dressing and gently toss to cover them. You cannot need any of the dressing, depending on the size of the cauliflower heads. As needed, wear. In a serving dish, spoon the salad and finish with more cheese and minced cilantro. Immediately serve. Cover and chill before served, to serve afterwards.

43 Keto Mexican Spaghetti Casserole

Servings: 8 | **Time:** 1 hr | **Difficulty:** Easy

Nutrients per serving: Calories: 365 kcal | Fat: 27 | Carbohydrates: 9g | Protein: 22g | Fiber: 2g

Ingredients

2 Tbsp. tomato paste

2 Tbsp. chili powder

2 oz. cream cheese softened

1/3 cup diced bell pepper

1/2 tsp. cumin

1/2 cup diced onion

1 spaghetti squash about 10.8 cups or 4 cups cooked

1 cup water

1 1/2 cups shredded medium cheddar divided

1 ½ tsp. salt divided

1 ½ tsp. garlic powder

5.4 cups ground beef or venison

¼ cup sliced green onion

Method

1. Preheat the oven to 400°F. Using a fork or knife to pierce the squash numerous times and microwave it for 3-4 minutes. Remove it gently from the oven, cut off the sides. Drizzle with avocado oil on the cut side, sprinkle with salt and put on a sheet pan lined with parchment, cut side down. For 30-45 minutes or until soft, roast. Roast time can depend on your squash's size.

2. Meanwhile, roast the beef or venison over medium heat in a large skillet with bell pepper, onion, garlic powder and half a teaspoon of salt. Continue cooking until the caramelization of the meat occurs and the vegetables are tender. Add the cumin and chili powder and simmer for an additional minute. Add the tomato paste, water, the rest of the salt and cook for 1-2 minutes or until the paste is thickened. Taste the mixture of chili and change the salt as needed. Stir in the cream cheese and 1 cup of the shredded cheese and remove from the sun. Stir until it is melted and thoroughly mixed in with the cheese.

3. Attach the spaghetti squash that has been prepared and toss to blend. Pour the mixture of chili and squash into a lightly greased saucepan, cover with the remaining cheese and bake for 15 minutes at 400 °F or until the cheese is melted and bubbly.

4. Top and eat soft with sliced green onions.

44 Keto Zucchini Gratin with Poblanos

Servings: 8 | **Time**: 25 mins | **Difficulty**: Easy

Nutrients per serving: Calories: 230 kcal | Fat: 20g | Carbohydrates: 6g | Protein: 7g | Fiber: 2g

Ingredients

½ tsp. garlic powder

¾ cup heavy cream

1 ¼ tsp. cumin

1 ¼ tsp. salt divided

1 ½ cup shredded Monterey Jack cheese or Pepper Jack divided

1 clove garlic

1 small onion diced

2 poblano peppers seeded and diced

2 Tbsp. sour cream

3 Tbsp. butter

4 zucchinis cut in half lengthwise and sliced

Method

1.   Preheat the oven to 400°F.

2.   Melt the butter, put the onion, poblano, 1⁄2 tsp. in a large oven-safe skillet over medium heat. Add salt and simmer for 5-7 minutes until tender. Connect the cumin and garlic and simmer for an additional minute. Stir in the sliced zucchini and season with 1⁄2 tsp. Continue to cook for another 5 minutes or until the zucchini is tender.

3.   Stir in the milk and simmer for an additional minute. Stir in 1 cup of cheese, sour cream, and the remaining 1⁄4 tsp. salt.

4.   Add the remaining cheese to the top and bake for 10-12 minutes or until bubbly. Switch the broiler on high and cook for 2-3 more minutes or until browned on top. Remove from the oven and let sit before serving for 5 minutes.

45   Keto Shrimp Etouffee with Crawfish

Servings: 4 | **Time:** 30 mins | **Difficulty:** Easy

Nutrients per serving: Calories: 427 kcal | Fat: 32g | Carbohydrates: 8g | Protein: 24g | Fiber: 3g

Ingredients

¼ cup sliced green onions

¼ tsp. cayenne pepper

½ cup heavy cream

½ tsp. pepper

½ tsp. salt

¾ cup diced onion

1 cup diced bell pepper

1 cup diced celery

1 cup shrimp or chicken stock

1 pound crawfish tails thawed

1 pound raw large shrimp peeled & deveined,

1 tsp. dried oregano

1 tsp. dried thyme

1 tsp. paprika

3 oz. cream cheese softened

4 cloves garlic finely chopped

4 Tbsp. butter

Method

1.　　Over medium heat in a large pan, add butter. Melt the butter and proceed to cook for 3-5 minutes or until the butter is finely browned, stirring regularly. For around 5-7 minutes, add the diced celery, onion, and pepper to the butter and proceed to cook until the onion is translucent and the vegetables begin to brown.

2.　　Mix the paprika, the oregano, the thyme, the peppers and the salt in a small bowl and put aside. Attach the vegetables to the minced garlic and simmer for another minute.

3.　　Apply the spice mixture to the vegetables and simmer, stirring continuously, for another minute. To blend, apply the stock to the veggie and spice mixture and whisk well. Simmer showed himself for 6-8 minutes. Apply the cream to the skillet and proceed to cook for a further 5-7 minutes or until the mixture is thickened and the back of the spoon is coated.

4.　　Add the crawfish and shrimp to the pan after the sauce has thickened. Cook for 2-3 minutes until the shrimp is thoroughly cooked. Remove the pan from the heat and swirl until it is thoroughly melted and mixed into the cream cheese.

5.　　Sprinkle over the top of the shrimp and crawfish with the green onions and garnish with chopped parsley if desired. Over steamed cauliflower rice, serve.

46 Keto Lemon & Garlic Grilled Chicken Quarters

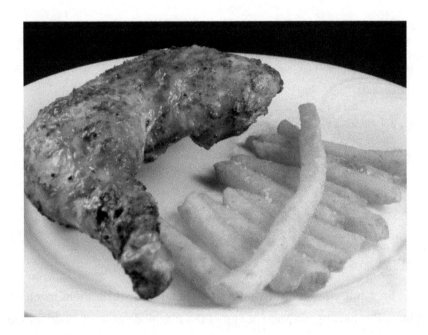

Servings: 8 | **Time:** 7 hrs | **Difficulty**: Easy

Nutrients per serving: Calories: 438 kcal | Fat: 34g | Carbohydrates: 1g | Protein: 31g

Ingredients

Garnish: Chopped Parsley & Lemon Wedges Fiesta Brand Lemon Pepper & Salt

14.4 cups chicken leg quarters about 4 quarters

10 cloves garlic smashed and roughly chopped

1/2 tsp. dried thyme crushed

1 cup fresh lemon juice

1 cup avocado oil

1 ½ Tbsp. salt

½ tsp. pepper

½ tsp. paprika

¼ tsp. onion powder

Method

1.   In a tub, combine the first 8 ingredients and whisk them together to combine. For basting, scrape 1/2 cup of the marinade and set aside for later. Divide the chicken into 2 ziptop bags and dump into each bag ½ of the remaining marinade. Let the air out of the bags and combine with the marinade to coat the chicken. Refrigerate for 6-8 hours while marinating, spinning the bags 2-3 times.

2.   Preheat the grill to 325°F or so. Remove and put the chicken from the bag on a sheet pan; discard the marinade. Lightly season the chicken with salt and lemon pepper. Grill covered for 20-25 minutes on the skin side up. Switch the chicken and grill for an extra 20-25 minutes or until finished, always basting the chicken with the marinade reserved. Sprinkle with minced parsley and serve with lemon wedges. Put the chicken on the serving platter.

47 Grilled Salmon with Cilantro Lime Crema

Servings: 4 | **Time:** 30 mins | **Difficulty:** Easy

Nutrients per serving: Calories: 380 kcal | Fat: 25.6g | Carbohydrates: 5.5g | Protein: 33.9g | Fiber: 0.5g

Ingredients

Olive oil

1 ½ pound salmon fillet cut into four pieces

For the Spice Rub:

1/8 tsp. Cayenne pepper

1 tsp. salt

1 ¼ tsp. dried oregano crushed

¾ tsp. garlic powder

½ tsp. paprika

½ tsp. chili powder

For the Cilantro Lime Crema:

1/8 tsp. cumin

1 Tbsp. fresh lime juice

1 Tbsp. chopped cilantro

1 clove garlic finely minced

¼ tsp. salt

¼ tsp. lime zest

¼ cup sour cream

¼ cup mayonnaise your favorite

Method

1.   For the Crema: Add all the ingredients for the cream in a small mixing bowl and stir to combine. Before serving, cover and refrigerate.

2.   Preheat to 350-400°F on your barbecue.

3.   Mix all the ingredients for the spice rub in a small bowl and mix well to combine. Drizzle the bits of salmon with olive oil and season the spice mixture liberally on both sides. Set the side of the salmon skin down on the hot barbecue. Cook on each side for about 8 minutes, turning once.

4.   To serve: drizzle the cream and sprinkle with minced cilantro over the grilled salmon. With new lime, serve.

48 Mexican Shredded Beef

Servings: 6 | **Time**: 1 hr 5 mins | **Difficulty**: Easy

Nutrients per serving: Calories: 421 kcal | Fat: 27g | Carbohydrates: 3g | Protein: 38g | Fiber: 1g

Ingredients

Salt Pepper & Garlic Powder

3 cloves garlic finely chopped

2.5 pound chuck roast

2 Tbsp. avocado oil

2 Tbsp. adobo sauce from the can of chipotles

2 chipotle peppers seeded and diced

1/2 onion diced

1 tsp. salt

1 tsp. garlic powder

1 tsp. chili powder

1 cup beef broth or stock

1 1/2 tsp. cumin

½ cup chopped bell pepper

Method

1.   By choosing the sauté setting and turning it up to heavy, preheat the Instant Pot. With salt, pepper and garlic powder, season the chuck roast on both sides. Once it's warmed, stir in the oil and add the roast. Sear for 4-5 minutes or until golden brown on either foot.

2.   Turn the heat off until the beef is seared and add the next 10 ingredients. Place the cap on the Instant pot and put the valve in the position of the seal. Cook on high pressure for 55 minutes and normal release for 20 minutes.

3.   Turn the valve gently so that any residual strain is removed and close the lid. Remove the beef from the liquid and put and shred it on a plate or tray. On the sauté setting, turn the Instant Pot back on high and bring the remaining liquid to a boil to minimize the pot. Simmer for about 10 minutes... there should be about 1-1⁄2 cups of liquid left. Carry the shredded beef back to the pot. Serve with diced coriander, new lime, pico de gallo and sliced avocado served with cauliflower rice!

49   Chipotle Lime Grilled Pork Chops

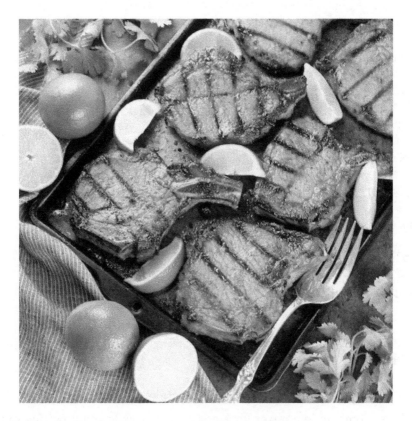

Servings: 6 | **Time:** 4 hrs 30 mins | **Difficulty:** Easy

Nutrients per serving: Calories: 317 kcal | Fat: 19g | Carbohydrates: 5g | Protein: 29g | Fiber: 1g

Ingredients

For the marinade:

Salt Pepper & Garlic Powder

6 pork ribeyes ¾" to 1" thick

6 cloves garlic finely minced

4 Tbsp. oil

2 tsp. Lakanto Monkfruit Sweetener golden or classic

2 chipotle peppers seeded

1 tsp. salt

1 tsp. onion powder

1 tsp. cumin

1 tsp lime zest

½ cup fresh lime juice

Method

1.   Mix all the marinade ingredients into a glass jar and shake well to combine. Combine in a mixer for a creamier marinade and a basting sauce. With ½ of the marinade, placed the pork chops in a ziptop bag. Remove from the air and cool for 4-6 hours.

2.   Preheat the grill to 450°F until preparing for grilling. From the marinade, cut the pork chops and season with salt, pepper and garlic powder on both sides. Place chops on a preheated grill and cook 5- 7 minutes on each side, basting chops sometimes during cooking with the reserved marinade. Depending on the chops' thickness, the grilling time can vary, and the internal temperature should be 160°F. Remove from the grill and serve as needed, with any leftover marinade.

50 Asian Inspired Ground Venison Lettuce Wraps

Servings: 8 | **Time:** 25 mins | **Difficulty:** Easy

Nutrients per serving: Calories: 158 kcal | Fat: 9g | Carbohydrates: 3g | Protein: 14g | Fiber: 0g

Ingredients

Garnish:

sliced green onions and chopped dry roasted salted peanuts

6 oz. cremini or white button mushrooms cleaned and diced in ¼" pieces

4 cloves garlic finely minced or grated

3 Tbsp. rice wine vinegar

3 Tbsp. gluten-free soy sauce or Tamari

2 tsp. sriracha hot sauce optional

2 Tbsp. natural smooth peanut butter

1/3 cup water

1/2 tsp. granulated garlic

1 tsp. salt

1 Tbsp. sesame oil

1 Tbsp. olive oil

1 Tbsp. Lakanto Monkfruit sweetener

1 Tbsp. fresh grated ginger

1 pound ground venison

1 head iceberg lettuce washed and separated into individual leaves

1 8 oz. can water chestnuts drained and diced

¼ cup sliced green onions

Method

1.   Combine the vinegar, soy sauce, sesame oil, peanut butter, sugar or a substitute, and the sriracha in a little dish. To mix and set aside, stir.

2.   Apply the olive oil and venison to the pan in a large skillet over medium-high heat and start browning. Season with 1 teaspoon. 1/2 tsp and salt. Powder and garlic. Add the sliced mushrooms, garlic, chestnuts, ginger, and green onions after 2-3 minutes, and begin to cook until the meat is brown and begins to caramelize. You should have several bits stuck to the bottom of the pan at this stage. Apply the water to the pan and stir, wiping off the bottom of the pan with all the caramelized pieces.

3.   Pour in the sauce that has been cooked and apply to the meat mixture. Continue to cook, stirring continuously, for another 2-3 minutes, until no liquid is left in the pan.

4.   Place about half a cup of the meat mixture in the middle of the lettuce leaf to serve. Cover with green onion diced and peanuts diced, roll up and enjoy!